Get the most out of this book!

Visit
www.mycorebalance.com/summer-2019
for guidance through the workout plan.

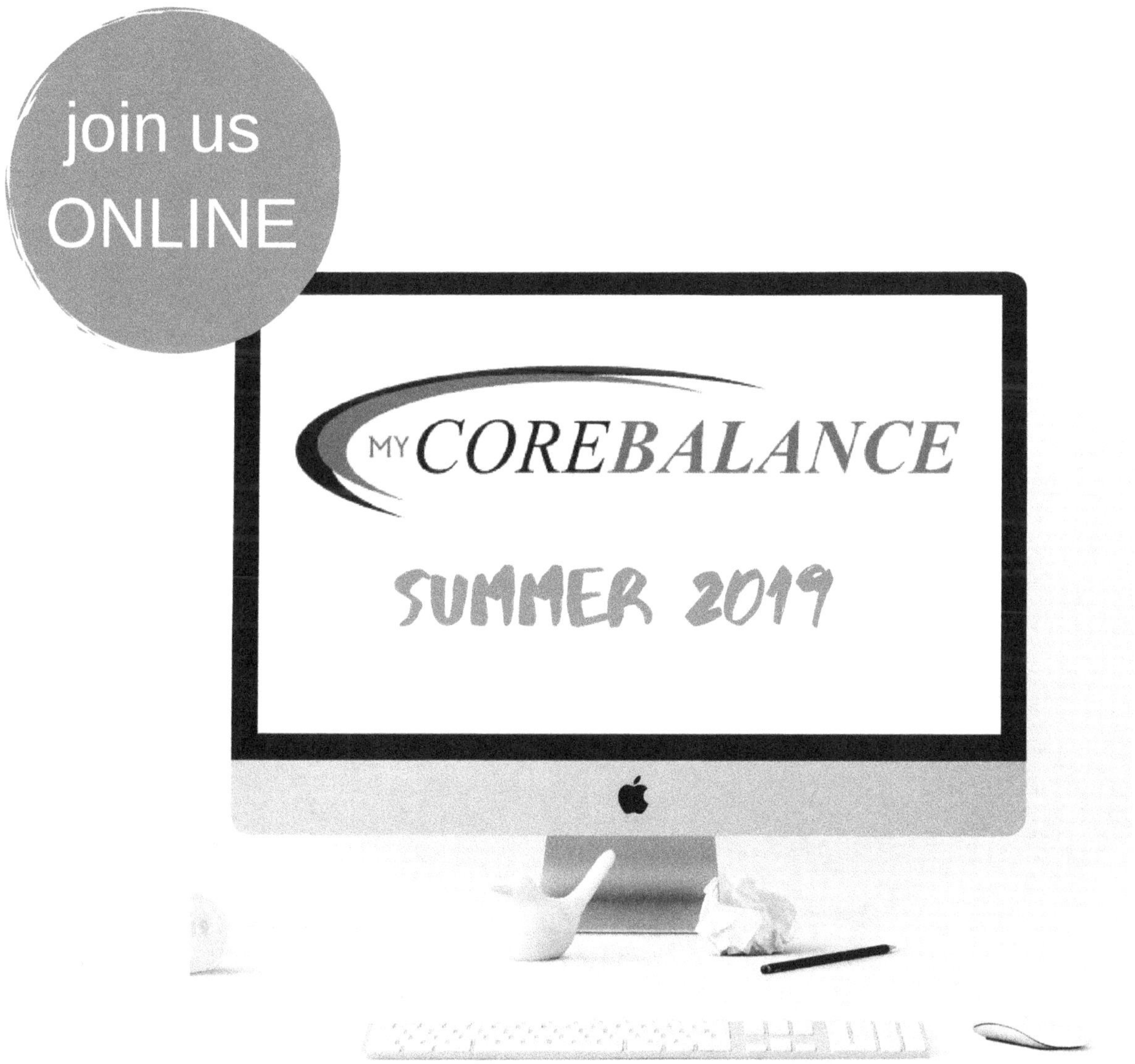

join us
ONLINE

MY COREBALANCE

SUMMER 2019

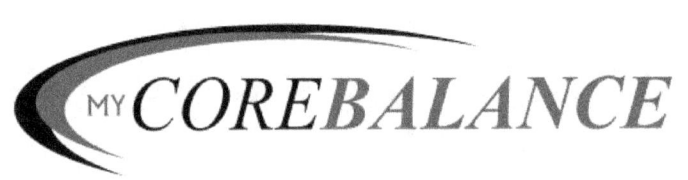

SUMMER

2019

Fitness Tracker

Chris Janke-Bueno

CONTENTS

WELCOME

Ahh, summer!

Hi,

I'm so excited to launch this new tracking book. You're holding the first edition of the quarterly My Core Balance training book.

This book came from your feedback. Seeing your progress is very motivating, telling you that you're going in the right direction.

FOCUS is extremely powerful. This book deliberately does not include a lot of things, because when we focus on just a few things, that's when we get great results.

If this is your first experience at My Core Balance,

WELCOME!

Thank you again for your participation. I look forward to helping you
achieve your fitness goals...
without injuring yourself.

In health,

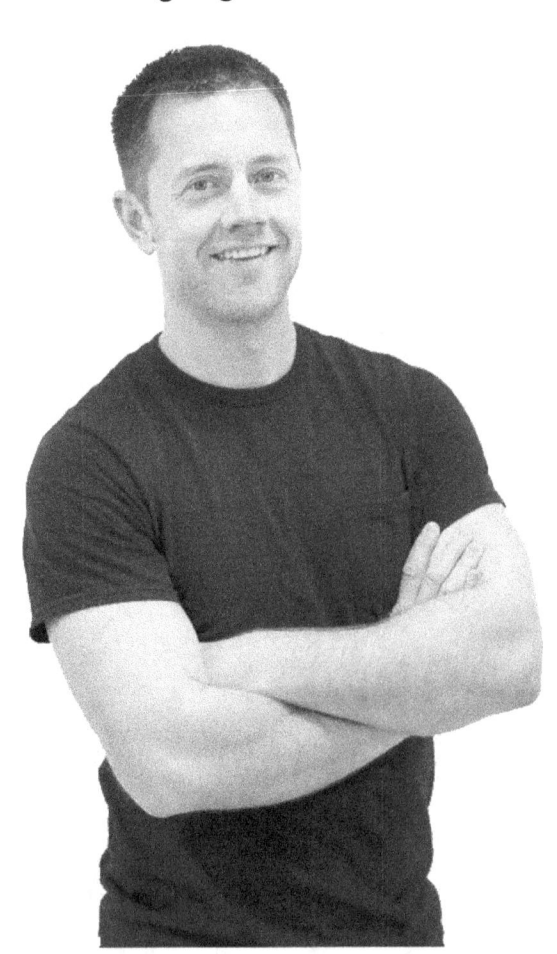

Chris JB

S.M.A.R.T. GOALS SUMMER 2019

What do you *really* want?

What is your big picture SPECIFIC goal?

How will you MEASURE that goal?

What ACTIONS will you consistently take?

Why? What's the REASON you want to achieve your goal?

How much TIME until you reach your big picture goal? Will it happen this quarter?

ASSESSMENT

Track your progress

Start	Goals	End
Weight _____	Weight _____	Weight _____
Body Fat %	Body Fat %	Body Fat %
_____	_____	_____
Chest _____	Chest _____	Chest _____
Waist _____	Waist _____	Waist _____
Upper Arm _____	Upper Arm _____	Upper Arm _____
Lower Arm _____	Lower Arm _____	Lower Arm _____
Thigh _____	Thigh _____	Thigh _____
Calf _____	Calf _____	Calf _____
Neck _____	Neck _____	Neck _____

ASSESSMENT

Track your progress

	Start	End
How is your energy level?		
Stress level?		
How much back pain do you have?		
How are you sleeping?		

5

WEEKLY SPLIT

Your Workout Schedule

Your "split" refers to how you divide up your week. This is done from a macro level. No details yet. Ask yourself, "how do I want to divide my week?" Be sure to include stretching, core, strength, cardio, and rest. Take into account the other big obligations in your life: work, family, social, etc.

MON

TUE

WED

THU

FRI

SAT

SUN

Your Daily Plan

Nutrition tracking has its place, but I've found that it can be more effective to create an "ideal day" and then work to try to reach that plan. Take a few minutes to write out what an ideal day looks like from a food perspective. If time, money, and eating out weren't issues, what's *your* perfect diet?
NOTE: you don't need to fill out all sections.

WAKE UP

BREAKFAST

SNACK

LUNCH

SNACK

DINNER

	Date								
90-90 with 2 Pillows									
Hands and Knees Elbow									
Curls									
Bird-Dog									
Twist Plank									
Overhead Wall Squat									
Superman									
Pullovers with Leg Raises									
Table Top									
Windmill									

Instructions: Track best time in boxes

M = Modification

X = Skip it!

Notes

Homework

CORE

Workout #2

	Date							
1-Leg Glute Bridges								
Hollow Body								
Side Plank Leg Raises								
Incline Close Flies								
Side Arm Circles								
Standing Rotator Cuff								
Table Top								
Inchworm								
Core Roll								

Instructions: Track best time in boxes

M = Modification

X = Skip it!

Notes

Homework

Date
Bridge with
Strap
90-90 with Ring
Hip Lift
Hip Twist
L Breakdancer
Inchworm
Superman
Back Bridge
Full Sit Ups

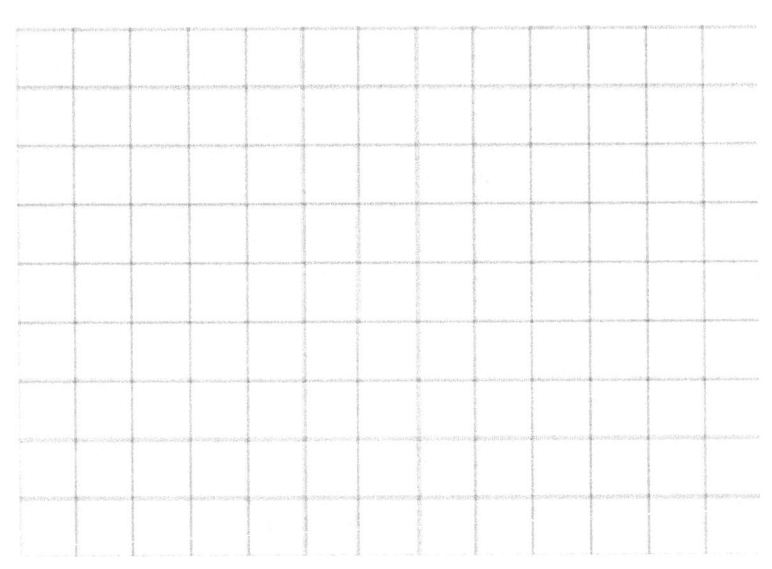

Instructions: Track best time in boxes
M = Modification
X = Skip it!

Notes

Homework

STRENGTH

Workout A

Date
Squat
Overhead Press
Dead Lift
Barbell Curls
Hanging Leg Raises
Weighted Windmill
Overhead Tricep
Extension

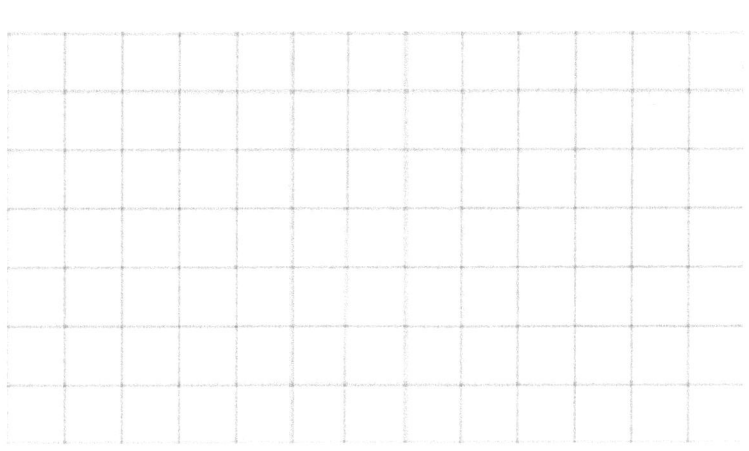

Instructions: 5 sets of 5 reps
Track best lift in boxes
M = Modification
X = Skip

Notes

Homework

STRENGTH

Workout B

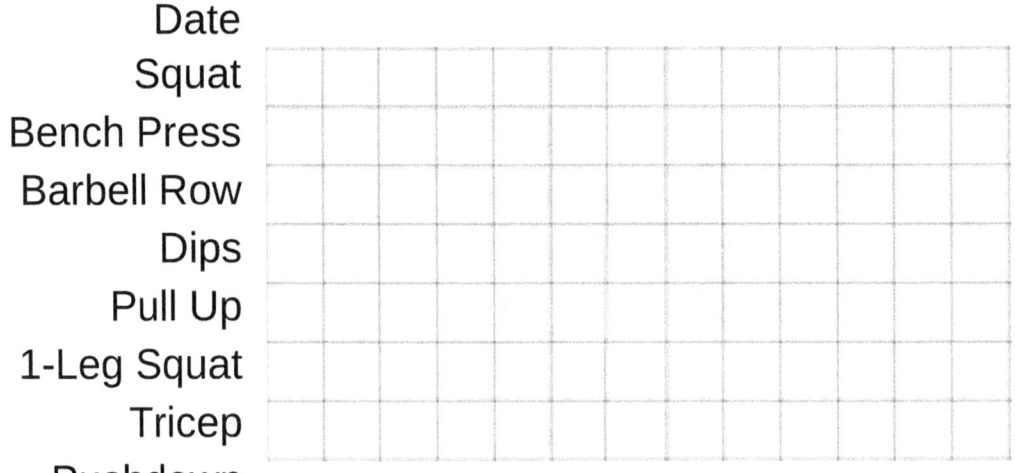

Date								
Squat								
Bench Press								
Barbell Row								
Dips								
Pull Up								
1-Leg Squat								
Tricep Pushdown								

Instructions: 5 sets of 5 reps

Track best lift in boxes

M = Modification

X = Skip

Notes

Homework

STRENGTH

Workout C

Date								
Turkish Get Up								
Static Full Sit-Up								
Presses								
Bent Squat								
Farmer's Walk								
Dumbbell Curls								
Supine Tricep								

Instructions: 5 sets of 5 reps

Track best lift in boxes

M = Modification

X = Skip

Notes

Homework

H.I.T.

High Intensity Interval Training

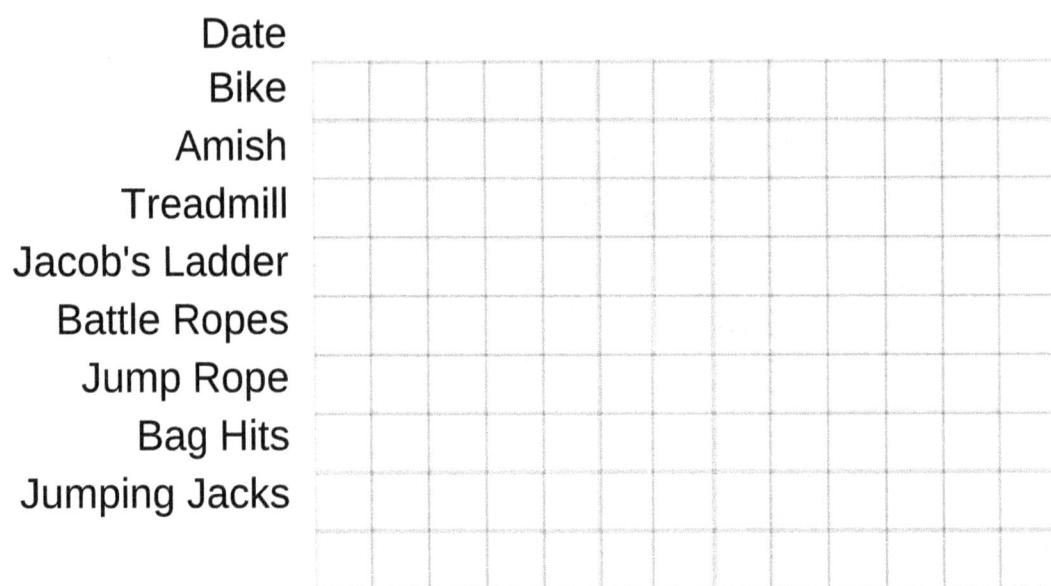

| Date |
| Bike |
| Amish |
| Treadmill |
| Jacob's Ladder |
| Battle Ropes |
| Jump Rope |
| Bag Hits |
| Jumping Jacks |

Instructions: Tabata - 20 sec work, 10 sec rest (8 times)
Track number of "8 packs" (1 to 5)

Notes

Homework

14

Low Intensity Steady State

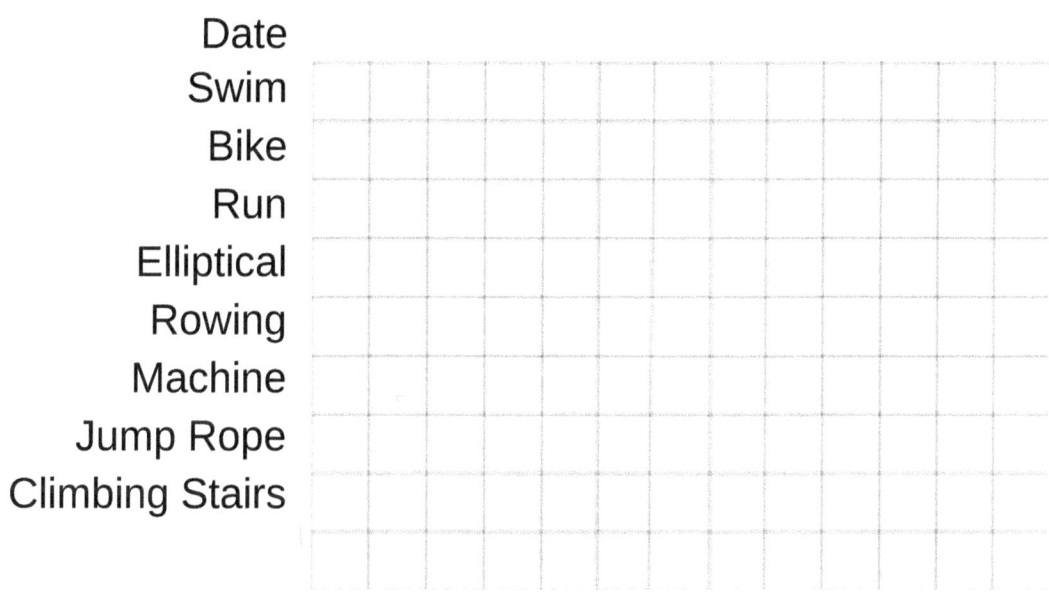

Date
Swim
Bike
Run
Elliptical
Rowing
Machine
Jump Rope
Climbing Stairs

Instructions: Moderate heart rate (talking pace)
Track number of minutes

Notes

Homework

Fitness Education

Pyramid of Health

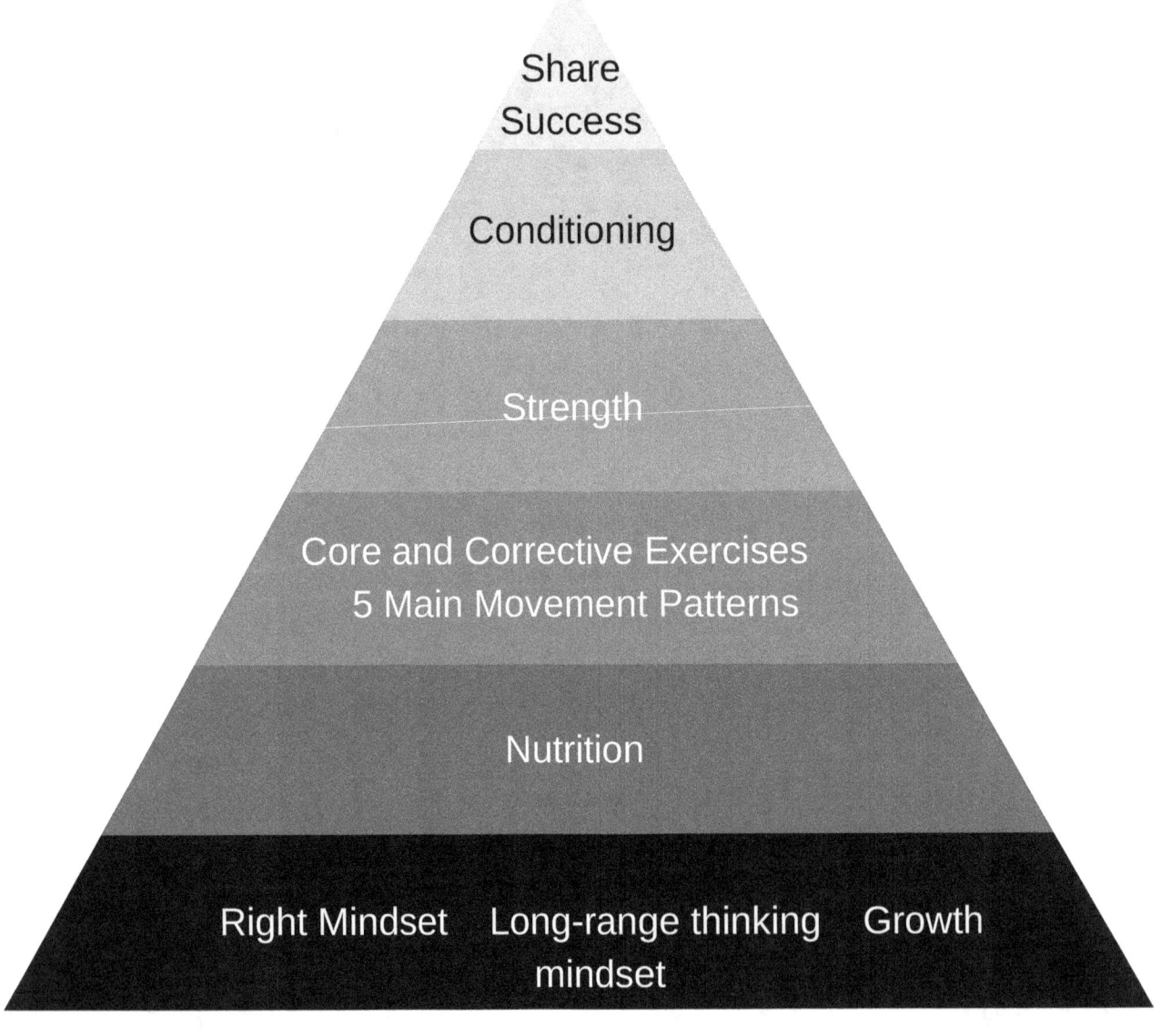

Are Your Hamstrings *Actually* Tight?

I was standing there in disbelief. I was watching this advanced yoga practitioner standing right in front of me. He showed me how he could touch his elbows to the floor without bending his knees. I have never in my life seen somebody with such flexible hamstrings.

After hearing his story, and how much yoga has helped him to calm down his mind, I asked him how I could help. It was his first appointment with me in my personal training studio.

His response sent my jaw to the floor. I couldn't believe it.

He wanted me to help him with his issue of...

Are you ready for this?

Tight hamstrings!

His number one complaint was that his hamstrings always felt tight.

Are you are surprised as I was? How can a man who is so obviously flexible have "tight" hamstrings?

Well, the answer is that he doesn't. His hamstrings are extremely flexible, in fact they are too flexible. But to him, they *felt* tight.

Upon further investigation, I determined that he has an anterior tilted pelvis. Because his hips are tilted forward, or anterior, the hamstrings are under a constant pull. So that feeling of hamstring tightness is actually the feeling that his hamstrings always at the end of the range of motion, stretching.

The solution for this particular client was to strengthen the hamstrings and abdominals. We also needed to stretch the hip flexors and quads.

Within a few weeks he stopped complaining of his hamstring tightness. He also lost a few inches of hamstring flexibility. However, he could still touch his hands to the floor very easily. And he was happy to lose a few inches of flexibility if it meant becoming pain-free.

Be careful of your body's tricks. You can't simply go based on *feeling* tight. You need to remember that the feeling might be there because the hamstrings are weak. Use the exercises as the assessment, and be open to change direction if your body sends you the wrong signals.

What changes do you need to make next quarter?

What worked well?

Did you reach your goal? Why or why not?

To purchase the next fitness tracker book, *Fall 2019*, visit
www.mycorebalance.com/fit-track

www.ingramcontent.com/pod-product-compliance
Lightning Source LLC
Chambersburg PA
CBHW080358290526
45791CB00009BA/2923